YOUR KNOWLEDGE HAS VALUE

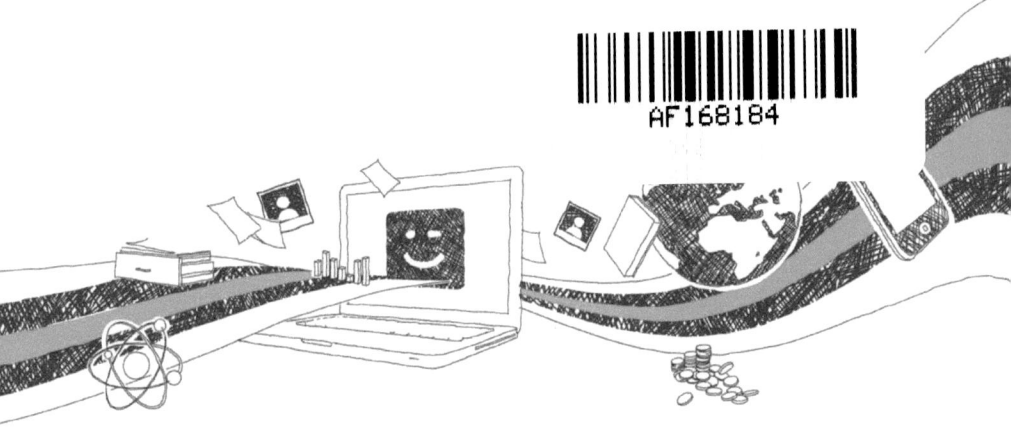
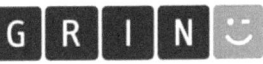

Bibliographic information published by the German National Library:

The German National Library lists this publication in the National Bibliography; detailed bibliographic data are available on the Internet at http://dnb.dnb.de .

Imprint:

Copyright © 2018 GRIN Verlag
Print and binding: Books on Demand GmbH, Norderstedt Germany
ISBN: 9783346069214

This book at GRIN:

https://www.grin.com/document/502225

Rimsha Khan

Diabetes Awareness Study in General Population of Punjab, Pakistan

GRIN Verlag

GRIN - Your knowledge has value

Since its foundation in 1998, GRIN has specialized in publishing academic texts by students, college teachers and other academics as e-book and printed book. The website www.grin.com is an ideal platform for presenting term papers, final papers, scientific essays, dissertations and specialist books.

Visit us on the internet:

http://www.grin.com/

http://www.facebook.com/grincom

http://www.twitter.com/grin_com

Diabetes Awareness Study in General Population of Punjab, Pakistan.

Project Report

by

Rimsha Khan

Department of Pharmacy Practice

Dedications

We dedicate our hard-work and all efforts to our loving

Parents

Who always pray for us and give us encouragement in every

situation

And also, to our honorable and hardworking teachers

Table of Contents

List of Tables

List of Figures

List of symbols and abbreviations

DM	Diabetes Mellitus
NIDDK	National institute of diabetes and digestion and kidney disease

Acknowledgments

I start in the Name of Allah, The Rehman, The Raheem, The Supreme and The Merciful. All thanks to Allah Almighty Who made me mentally and physically fit and enabled me in pursuing the Hadith of the Holy Prophet Hazrat Muhammad (P.B.U.H) *"The seeking of knowledge is obligatory for every Muslim." – (Al-Tirmidhi, Hadith 74).*

I express my gratitude to my research supervisor **Dr. Muhammad Fawad Rasool**, whose kind support and guidance keep me on track to accomplish the task with an overwhelming success. In addition, the authors would like to thanks Dr. Nasir Kalam for their suggestion and assistance in completing the project report writing.

My acknowledgement goes to all the faculty and staff members of the Department of Pharmacy Bahauddin Zakariya University. I would also like to extend my deepest thanks to all academic colleagues Bahauddin Zakariya University.

Abstract

Background: Diabetes is a chronic, metabolic disease characterized by high blood sugar levels. To fall into the diabetic category, IGT the impaired glucose levels of a person are in the range of 140 to 199 mg/dL at two-hours after an OGTT. In IFG that is impaired fasting glucose the range is 110 to 125 mg/ dL. One can have an idea of the prevalence of diabetes by the fact that the population affected by diabetes worldwide has gone from 108 million to 422 million from 1980 to 2014.

Objective: The aim of the study was to determine the awareness of the people of Punjab, Pakistan about the basic knowledge of Diabetes. The reason for this was because of the increasing prevalence and complications of Diabetes and associated diseases.

Methods: The study settings were Bahauddin Zakariya University, Multan, Al shifa pharmacy Multan, Clinic. An online survey was also conducted. The sample size was 752 and the research tool used was a questionnaire having questions for knowledge of diabetes. The time of data collection was January 2018 to April 2018. Data was analyzed by Microsoft excel 2010 and SPSS 20.

Results: 15.9% of the participants did not have any concept of diabetes. 34% said the disease is contagious and 61.7% said the disease is curable although neither it is contagious nor curable. Hence, it can be said that the female participants had a better knowledge about the factors leading to the development of diabetes. Out of the 529 patients who had a diabetic in their family 359 participants were aware of all of the factors while only 157 out of 259 participants without a diabetic in their family knew all of the given factors contribute to diabetes.

Conclusion: The study showed that people with a diabetic in their family had better knowledge about the disease as compared to the people who don't. This shows that the public needs to be educated from time to time about the basics, factors, underlying causes, prevention, cure & complications associated with diabetes. Interactive seminars for general public especially students about diabetes & diabetes awareness Educational programs in institutes are the need of the hou

Introduction

Diabetes in its simple definition is elevated blood sugar level which may lead to different complications. Diabetes mellitus is a disorder which is genetic; the person suffers from hyperglycemia, vascular disorder and neuropathy (Fajans, 1971). Diabetes is a chronic disorder that affects the overall quality of life no matter how early the stage of the disease is. It worsens the health with the passage of time. It does not only affect the blood but as time passes, the person is prone to various kinds of infections, weakness, decreased immunity, not to forget its hazardous effects on most of our organs including the eyes, the nervous system, both kidneys, nervous system, hands and feet, even the brain and the heart. The most common complications associated with diabetes are nephropathy & neuropathy along with many others. Continuously elevated blood sugar levels decreases the body's various abilities including peripheral nerves and immune responses which lead to numbness as well as lowering the ability of the body to fight wounds.

Types:

Diabetes is of various types classified according to age on onset, inheritance, production of insulin, production of other hormones in the body, diabetes related and confined only to pregnancy etc. but commonly classified either as type 1 or type 2 diabetics. Type 1 diabetes starts often in the early childhood whilst Type 2 diabetes is diabetes mellitus which often develops in late age stages. The reason & mechanism of both type of diabetes are totally different. In type 1 diabetes, person has no insulin secretion while in type 2, the person is deficient of insulin or is resistant to its affects or both deficient in production and resistant to its actions (Association, 2011). Type 2 diabetes may involve factors like genetic, obesity, physical work and diet. Type 2 diabetes is the most common diabetes prevailing in the world right now. You can't treat it but you can live a healthy life by managing it. Management is the only solution to avoid diabetes related complications.

Prevalence:

One can have an idea of the prevalence of diabetes by the fact that the population affected by diabetes worldwide has gone from 108 million to 422 million from 1980 to 2014 (World Health Organization, 2014). 12.8% global deaths were attributed for deaths of ages between 20-79. According to data collection of 2015, 7.2% U.S. population have developed known diabetes, which has 132,000 children & young adults, only 5% diabetic persons have been calculated to have type 1 diabetes (Centers for Disease Control and Prevention, 2017). And when we talk about Pakistan, the estimation of diabetes affected individuals in 2040 will get doubled as compared to 2015 (International Diabetes Federation, 2017).This is an extremely alarming situation because people are just unaware of the fact how diabetes has developed its roots in the society. Furthermore, diabetes mellitus, especially type 2 diabetes is a preventable disease, and hence awareness of diabetes, how it is caused and how can it be prevented is really important as it can lead to decrease in the rates of prevalence of diabetes in our society. If the factors leading to diabetes do not get controlled, it will surely be the leading cause of deaths in future.

The only solution as already mentioned is actually preventing the disease. One can prevent diabetes type 2 but one cannot prevent type 1 diabetes. Type 2 diabetes prevention is the need of the hour and in order to achieve that, the population needs to be educated. If people are more aware of the factors which lead to diabetes, they can prevent the disease progression. But there are some factors that can't be controlled and among them are geographic, genetic as well as age type of factors (International Diabetes Federation, 2017). Major prevention recommendations involve walk, exercise, healthy diet (water or tea over juices, vegetables, nuts, and unsaturated fats), regular checkups as well as weight control. Gestational diabetes (which means diabetes during pregnancy) and prediabetes (people who are at a high risk for developing diabetes) are often related to have diabetes in those persons in future. As well as other diseases in an individual may lead to diabetes or will exaggerate the situation. For example high blood pressure is highly associated with the development of diabetes type 2. According to CDC report on national diabetes statistics, 73.6% diabetics have high blood pressure, 66.9% have dyslipidemia or high cholesterol issue, 15.9% have smoking in their routine, 87.5% are obese, 36.5% have kidney disease & 40.8% are physically inactive (International Diabetes Federation, 2017). Already diabetic patients are prone to develop nephropathy, retinopathy, cardio vascular problems, Alzheimer, teeth problems & above all is diabetic foot. Diabetics often develop neuropathy which causes numbness and patients don't often even realize if they have got an infection or wound somewhere. This often leads to serious infections and the major damage is in the form of diabetic foot.

The management of diabetes is done by medications, but many can be managed with exercise and diet control only. There are various classes of drugs available to manage the disease. Some of them are sulphonyl ureas, biguanides, Thiazolidinediones, GLP-1 analogues, DPP4 inhibitors & Insulins. Sulphonyl ureas include tolbutamide, glimepiride, glyburide & glipizide etc. Biguanides include mainly metformin, Thiazolidinediones include pioglitazone & rosiglitazone, Alpha glucosidase inhibitors include Acarbose, Meglitinides include nateglinide, DPP4 inhibitors include linagliptin, sitagliptin & saxagliptin, Bile acid sequestrant include colesevelam, Dopamine agonist include bromocriptine, GLP-1 receptor agonists include exenatide, liraglutide, pramlintide & albiglutide. Insulins include short acting, intermediate acting, long acting & combination of these insulins. For type 1 diabetes, only insulin is required for the survival as other drugs will not help unless the body is producing insulin so lack of insulin production can only be corrected via exogenous insulin (externally administered into the body). Rapid acting insulin includes lispro and aspart etc. Short acting insulins include regular & velosulin. Intermediate acting insulins include NPH & Lente. Long acting insulins include ultralente, glargine, and detemir. Pre-mixed insulins include Humulin 70/30, Novolin 70/30, Novolog 70/30, Humulin 50/50, and Humalog 75/25.

For the management of diabetes, follow ABCs which means A1c level, blood pressure, cholesterol & smoking, respectively (National Institute of Diabetes and Digestive and Kidney Diseases). The patients with diabetes need to manage their high blood pressure, quit smoking, lower their cholesterol levels & normalize their A1c in ideal situations and this is the goal of therapy as well.

Controlling the disease will improve the quality of life; decrease morbidity rate and will eventually decrease mortality. But how is one supposed to prevent or manage when the person isn't even aware of the risk factors, causes, medications and everything associated with diabetes, so what needs to be emphasized is to aware general public.

Literature Review

Awareness and knowledge of diabetes in Chennai:

25% of the Chennai population didn't know what diabetes is. 11.9% of the participants knew about the risk factors like obesity and physical inactivity are causing the disease prevalence. 19% knew that this disease can cause further complications as well. The conclusion of the study was that India lacks the awareness of diabetes which is the need of the hour. (Mohan et al., 2005).

Diabetes knowledge in Kuwaiti adults:

Due to high illiteracy rate, the awareness of diabetes is very low. Poor socio-economic class also had a lower sense of knowledge. Even the diabetes affected patients had a lower level of awareness (Al-Adsani et al., 2009).

There have been various researches conducted on the knowledge & awareness of diabetes in the general population. According to the CDC (2008), overweight & less physical activity in young adults and children has caused an increased ratio of type 2 diabetes. A lot of Literature review has been done in the study which was done in 2016 by Nyamutsamba which tells about the risk factors awareness associated with diabetes (Nyamutsamba, 2016).

Aim of the study:

Pakistan is a developing country and we still need these basic studies in order to determine the root cause of many problems. The aim of the study was to determine the awareness of the people of Punjab, Pakistan about the basic knowledge of Diabetes. The reason for this was because of the increasing prevalence and complications of Diabetes and associated diseases (Zuhaid et al., 2012).

Materials and Methods

The purpose of this study was to determine the knowledge of diabetes in general population of Southern Punjab, Pakistan. The research methodology applied involves study type, study settings, sample size, research tool, Inclusion/Exclusion criteria, Statistical analysis tool and statistical formulas.

Study Type:

The design used in the research study is known as study type. There are various type and designs for research studies. Major among them are descriptive, experimental, co-relational, semi experimental, review, meta-analytical etc. The research design utilized for this diabetes awareness study was descriptive one. The descriptive design is the design which is rather systematic and gives facts, observations and characteristics about the population used as sample. Survey type of descriptive analysis was the mode of study. There are two types of study methods that can be used in a survey and following is the description of two types i.e. longitudinal study and cross sectional study. Longitudinal study is a study method in which same population group is studied but for a long period of time because this method is chosen when sequence of events in a population group is to be studied. The only disadvantage of this method is that it cannot be used in studies that needed to be done in a short period of time. In cross sectional study method data from different groups of a population is obtained. Even comparisons can be made of different variables. Moreover this study method required short time because it's not necessary to see the sequence of events in such surveys. This survey was also done using cross-sectional study method because the data was collected from university students, outdoor patients and general public and some of the data was also collected using an online questionnaire.

Study Settings:

The study settings are the area, place or the specific environment where a research is actually conducted. The study settings for this diabetes awareness study were various. These are Bahauddin Zakariya University, Multan, AL-shifa pharmacy, clinic and also through an online survey questionnaire. Day scholar students as well as hostellites of Bahauddin Zakariya University, Multan were involved in the data collection. Out-door patients and care takers were involved in data collection through AL-shifa pharmacy. Data was also taken from patients at a clinic setting. The online survey was done through questionnaire on google.docx and general public mostly from Punjab (and especially southern Punjab) of Pakistan were involved for the online survey.

Sampling Method

Different types of sampling methods are used in surveys and using these methods data is collected from the target population. Before starting a study, considering the target of attaining data from the population a method is selected this will be in favor of data collection. The types of sampling methods that can be used in a survey can be described as random, stratified, systematic, purposive, quota and convenient.

Random sampling techniques data is collected randomly from the population and in this sampling method there is no target population and anyone can be a part of that survey. Equal chances of being selected for each individual are a possibility. Stratified sampling is a sampling technique in which the individuals are made the subject of study in such a way that they must have same attributes like selecting people which have a common profession e.g. teachers, students etc. the chances of error in this sampling technique is way less than the Random sampling. Systematic sampling method in which an n number is chosen and while selecting the participants of the survey, every nth person is selected. To decide an n number is upon you and it can be any number. For example, if an n number 10 is decided in a survey, every nth (10th), 2nth (20th), 3nth (30th) and so on persons can participate in that survey. Purposive type of sampling method, a criterion is made and every person of population that fulfills those criteria is included for the study. The only disadvantage of this method is that one have to be confident enough that the people from population which meets the criteria will also be willing to participate in that survey. Convenient type of sampling, people which are willing to participate are made the subjects of that study. Any available individual can be selected to collect the data. The sampling method used in this study was Convenient

6

sampling because all the subjects which participated did it willingly, they consented to participate in the study by filling a structured questionnaire. Even for the online data collection, a google.docx link was given to the public. Anyone who willed to participate filled the survey. Quota Sampling method of sampling in which one can see similarity in between convenient and stratified sampling methods. In this method, sub sets are made and only people who will to participate, fill the questionnaire for the survey.

Sample Size:

The data collection was done from the time of January 2018 to April 2018. During this, data was collected from university students, outdoor patients & online public. Hence general public was involved. A total of 752 persons were involved for the data collection. Hence, the sample size was of 752. Out of these 752, 390 individuals participated through online survey while 100 outdoor patients participated in this study. 200 participants were from hostels of Bahauddin Zakariya University and the rest 62 participants were the students of Bahauddin Zakariya University.

Research Tool:

Research tool was a questionnaire. As the mode of study was descriptive analysis and survey methods are usually used to collect the descriptive data, the survey questionnaire was distributed to the general public and the same was online survey questionnaire consisted total of 14 number of questions was made available on google.docx. It consisted of demographic data of the participants involved including name, gender, age, city, marital status, socio economic status and presence of any major disease in the family. The questions included in the questionnaire were of both types i.e. open ended and closed ended questions. Major Key questions included concept about diabetes, organs affected, onset, risk factors involved in progression of disease. The knowledge about control, contagiousness, curability and preventability of the disease were also checked. Also if someone has diabetes in their family, they had to mention it.

The Questionnaire included following questions:

Patient's Name: _____

Marital Status: _____

Gender: Male/Female

Age: _____

Weight: _____

Height: _____

BMI: _____

Socio economic status: _____

Monthly Income: _____

Nature of Occupation: _____

Any Major disease in family: _____

1- Do you know what diabetes is? (Yes, No)
2- Diabetes is a condition that affects? (Heart, Cholesterol, Iron or Blood Sugar)
3- In diabetes, what is deficient? (Cholesterol, Insulin, Glucagon or Fats)
4- What organ is affected by diabetes? (Eyes, Feet, Kidneys, Fingers or All of the above)
5- Can diabetes lead to other disease? (Yes, No)
6- Can diabetes be controlled by? (Diet, Exercise, Controlling weight or All of the above)
7- Is diabetes contagious? (Yes, No)
8- Is diabetes preventable? (Yes, No)
9- Is diabetes curable? (Yes, No)
10- Can the onset of diabetes be delayed? (Yes, No)

11- What factors contribute to diabetes? (Obesity, Family History, Hormonal disorders or All of the above)

12- Insulin is a hormone that regulates? (Blood sugar, Cholesterol, Blood pressure, Don't know)

13- Do you think that more people are being affected by diabetes? Yes, No, Don't know)

14- Is there anyone in your family with diabetes? (Yes, No)

Inclusion and Exclusion criteria:

The inclusion criteria mean the limits or boundaries that allow the researcher to involve participants lying only in that region or limit. Exclusion criteria mean the boundary which defines that whoever is in the region isn't able to participate in that very research for which the criteria were set. After the data analyzing, it is checked whether the participants are in the exclusion criteria or not. In this survey there were no such inclusion and exclusion criteria except the geographical background for this study. People of Punjab, Pakistan were included in the study. Except this, without any discrimination anyone from general public regardless of their age, marital status, gender etc. was included. There was no compulsion for being a person to be diabetic or to have someone in family as a diabetic. Normal individuals as well as patients of any disease were welcome to fill the questionnaire. Hence, there was no exclusion or inclusion criteria except the local boundaries set as public of Punjab. The inclusion criteria were:

a. Patients with a geographical background of Southern Punjab, Pakistan.

b. Age group for the participants was 18 to 80 years.

c. Patients with and without Diabetes mellitus.

d. Patients with and without any other disease.

The exclusion criteria were:

a) People belonging to other areas of Pakistan.

b) People of age group below 18 and above 80.

9

Statistical Analysis Tool:

In carrying out a study statistical methods are involved. The statistical analysis tools are the tools used to analyze the data collected for research purposes and drawing meaningful reporting and interpretations from the data for result purposes. For this study, Microsoft Excel 2013 & SPSS 20 were used. Data was entered one by one in to the Microsoft excel & after making a spread sheet, the data was analyzed through SPSS 20. In SPSS, the data was encoded and the limits for variables were defined. Then the necessary tests were applied and results were calculated.

Statistical Formulas:

The statistical formulas are the formulas applied to analyze the data and to collect the results. Statistical formulas are often applied to co-relate two or even more factors or variables provided in the given data. For diabetes awareness study, the data was collected from general public through the questionnaire and then a spread sheet on Microsoft excel was formed, after that the SPSS was used to calculate the results as well as co-relations between factors or variables. The calculation of results and co-relations was done through applying some statistical formulas and tests. First of all, all the data was coded and then frequency was calculated. After that co-relations were found between variables like risk factors and number of females and males having the knowledge about it. Correlation in between family diabetes and knowledge of participants was also checked through SPSS 20.

Results

After collecting the data,the answers of all the participants of the survey were analysed statistically. This was done with the help of the analyzing tool software SPSS 25.0. The survey shows that 88.1 % (666) of the participants of the survey had a concept of diabetes while 11.1 % (84)of the participants did not have any idea about the disease. 84.1 % (635) of the participants knew that the disease affects only the blood sugar of the person who has it but 15.9 % (120) correctly answered that the disease effects other conditions such as cholesterol,iron and the heart. 81.6 % (617) knew the insulin is deficient in diabetes while 18.3 % answered that insulin effects other things like glucagon,cholesterol or fats in the body. Comparing the stats gender wise, out of 243 male participants, 151(61.1%) knew that factors precipitating diabetes a combination of obesity,family history and hormonal disorders while 92(37.8%) of the male participants considered only one of these three factors to predispose a person to diabetes.On the other hand, out of the the 514 female participants,366 (71.2 %) knew that all three factors can lead to diabetes while 148 (28.7 %) thought it was only one of these factors.

Table 3.1: Awareness of diabetes among general population

Awareness of Diabetes		n (%)
Do you know what diabetes is?	88.1 answered Yes	11.1 answered No
Diabetes is a condition that affects?	84.1 knew it affects blood sugar	15.9 chose the other options
Is Diabetes contagious?	65 answered that it is not	34.4 answered otherwise
Is Diabetes Curable?	38.3 said that it is not curable	61.7 answered that it is
What factors contribute to diabetes?	61.1 males anf 71.2 females knew about all the factors	37.8 males and 28.7 females considered only one of these
Do you think that more people are being affected by diabetes?	86.4 thought that more people are being affected by diabetes	13.6 answered otherwise

11

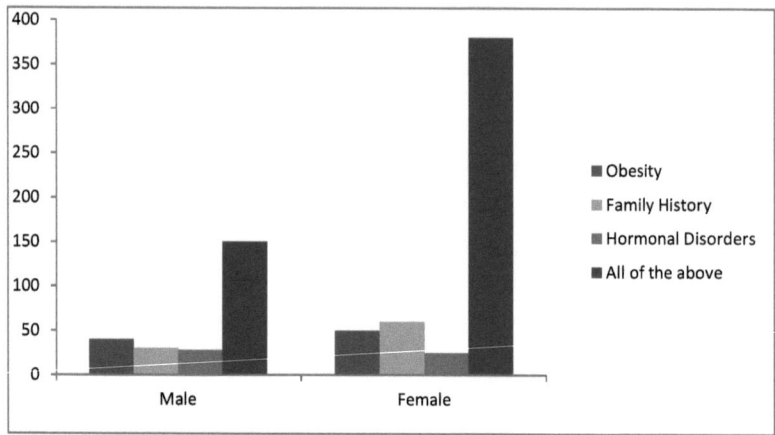

Fig 3.1 Co-relation of factors with the male and female population

From the above summary, it can be safely said that the female participants had a better knowledge about the factors leading to the development of diabetes as compared to the male counterparts that participated in the survey.

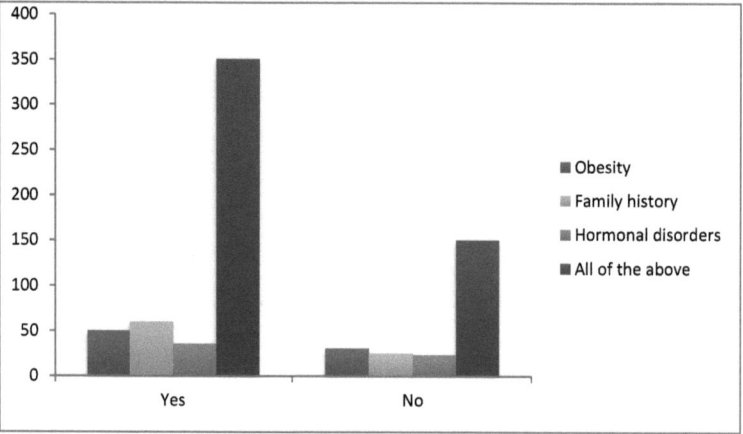

Fig 3.2 Co-relation of family DM with the knowledge of participants

Out of the 529 participants who had a diabetic patient in their family, 359 participants were aware of all of the factors while only 157 out of 259 participants who did not have a diabetic relative in their family knew all of the given factors contribute to diabetes.

Discussion

Diabetes awareness study in general population is such a basic thing for the research purposes in the vast field of diabetes but when it comes to patient knowledge, one can easily be surprised that even the disease has prevailed all over the world with such a high occurrence rate, people are still unaware of the facts and factors associated with the disease. This is not only common in the people who are affected by diabetes but there is also a high ratio of individuals suffering from diabetes and either they don't know or if they know, they don't know about the risk factors and prevention rules to avoid the progression of disease and its major complications. All this has created an alarming scenario.

General Knowledge of Diabetes:

From the above given results, it can easily be checked that 11.1% of the sample population didn't know all together that what is diabetes. 15.9% of the participants answered wrong about the basic concept of diabetes. Hence, 15.9% did not actually know what diabetes is. Although 15.9% may look insignificant but when a population who has almost the prevalence ratio of 1:7, it automatically looks significant, in fact alarming. (The diabetes awareness survey of Pakistan 2017) The general public is all set to be the preyed but what's actually happening, public is still lying in the world of misconception. In countries like under developed or developing countries, the awareness is even at a lesser ratio. A study was conducted in rural Tamaka, Kolar and it showed that more than seventy percent of the participants didn't know much about diabetes, They will not follow a diet plan if they are suggested with one. Hence it shows diabetes knowledge in general population is lower(Muninarayana et al., 2010).

Nature of Disease:

A few questions were trick questions to actually test the knowledge of participants. The participants were asked about the contagiousness of the disease. Contagious disease means a transferrable disease by touch. 34.3% answered, yes; it is contagious even though the disease is not contagious at all. This shows the lesser sense of knowledge about the diabetes of the participating individuals. The next thing with a surprising result is about the curability of the disease. 61.7% answered that it is curable. Although diabetes is not curable, it is actually a disorder and that is why it can be managed not cured, just like hypertension. 61.7% is such a high ratio of the participants

13

who think the disease has a cure. Once you are into diabetes, it is not going to leave you, you can improve quality of life, decrease the chances of complications associated with the disease but you can't simply avoid it.

Risk Factors:

37.8% males and 28.7% females did not have any idea that how many factors are actually related to diabetes. Diabetes is a disease which gets worsen by the factors involved. The factors are obesity, physical inactivity, exercise, diet, routine screening and genetic. The participants did not mostly know about the factors which are actually related to the disease. Factors act like a root for the disease progression. Routine medical screening for the high risk individuals is essential for improving the life span and quality of life. Diet is the key controlling factor as well as exercise. People need to be educated in this regard that medicines will not help if life style can't be changed.

Prevalence:

Respondents showed that most of them knew diabetes is prevailing these days. 13.6% answered otherwise. The prevalence of diabetes can be assumed by the fact that 366 million people will be affected by diabetes in 2030 and it is not even depending on obesity, instead it is being called as diabetes epidemic. (Wild et al., 2004)

Co-relation of Gender with the Knowledge of Risk Factors:

The co-relation results showed that females knew a lot more than males. This may be due to many reasons, mostly the diabetic or any other patient in a family is in care of the females of the house in Pakistan, and they might have a better sense of the disease progression than the males who seem to have a lower rate of knowledge. Another factor which may be involved is due to the higher population of females as compared to males in Pakistan.

Co-relation of Family Diabetes with the Knowledge of Participants:

The co-relation of family diabetes with the knowledge of people was also checked and it showed that a better sense of knowledge is associated with the diabetic in the family. Although it wasn't even much, but still as compared to the ones who didn't have a diabetic in their family, they knew more. A study was conducted in Pakistan relating to the knowledge of physicians about diabetes and it was a surprising result to see that Federal Capital Area physicians had knowledge of 54% and overall 62% had complete knowledge about diabetes. Hence, even doctors are at this stage of awareness when they deal with all type of patients as the participants in the study were family physicians (Shera et al., 2002). The people with a diabetic in their family may have a better knowledge but not every time.

Conclusion:

It can be deduced from this study that people with a diabetic patient in their family had better knowledge about the disease as compared to the people who do not have a diabetic family member. Hence it shows that mostly, only those people know about this dangerous and highly prevalent disease that has either been directly or indirectly affected by it. This clearly reflects that either there is no program in our society that is trying to create awareness about diabetes and its control and prevention or that the program is not successful enough yet. It has already been emphasized that the public needs to be educated from time to time about the basics, factors, underlying causes, prevention, cure & complications associated with diabetes. We need to utilize all sources of communication and all platforms to help bring this important issue to light. Educational programs on television, awareness campaigns via Facebook and other social networking sites, different workshops, interactive seminars for general public & Educational programs in educational institutes will help a long way in creating public awareness. Print media can also play its part by printing pamphlets and brochures about diabetes control and prevention. But the single most important factor that the society can benefit the most from is from doctors and healthcare providers to educate and council the masses about diabetes. Healthcare providers have access to not only diabetics or pre diabetics but patients with other diseases too and hence they can and should educate every single one of their patients about the hazards, warning signs, prevention, early detection and management of diabetes.

Bibliography:

AL-ADSANI, A. M. S., MOUSSA, M. A. A., AL-JASEM, L. I., ABDELLA, N. A. & AL-HAMAD, N. M. 2009. The level and determinants of diabetes knowledge in Kuwaiti adults with type 2 diabetes. *Diabetes & Metabolism,* 35, 121-128.

ASSOCIATION, A. D. 2011. Diabetes basics.

CENTERS FOR DISEASE CONTROL AND PREVENTION. 2017. *National Diabetes Statistics Report* [Online]. Available: https://www.cdc.gov/diabetes/pdfs/data/statistics/national-diabetes-statistics-report.pdf [Accessed 25 June 2018].

FAJANS, S. S. 1971. What is Diabetes?: Definition, Diagnosis, and Course. *Medical Clinics of North America,* 55, 793-805.

INTERNATIONAL DIABETES FEDERATION. 2017. *IDF diabetes atlas -18 edition* [Online]. Available: http://www.diabetesatlas.org/ [Accessed 25 june 2018].

MOHAN, D., RAJ, D., SHANTHIRANI, C., DATTA, M., UNWIN, N., KAPUR, A. & MOHAN, V. 2005. Awareness and knowledge of diabetes in Chennai-the Chennai urban rural epidemiology study [CURES-9]. *Japi,* 53, 283-287.

MUNINARAYANA, C., BALACHANDRA, G., HIREMATH, S., IYENGAR, K. & ANIL, N. 2010. Prevalence and awareness regarding diabetes mellitus in rural Tamaka, Kolar. *International journal of diabetes in developing countries,* 30, 18.

NATIONAL INSTITUTE OF DIABETES AND DIGESTIVE AND KIDNEY DISEASES. *What is diabetes* [Online]. Available: https://www.niddk.nih.gov/health-information/diabetes/overview/what-is-diabetes [Accessed 24 June 2018].

NYAMUTSAMBA, H. 2016. Relationship between knowledge levels of high active antiretroviral therapy (HAART) and adherence levels of HAART among HIV positive pregnant women aged 15 to 49 years attending antenatal care at Marondera provincial hospital, Family Child Health department, Zimbabwe.

SHERA, A., JAWAD, F. & BASIT, A. 2002. Diabetes related knowledge, attitude, and practices of family physicians in Pakistan. *Journal of Pakistan MedicalAssociation (JPMA).*

WILD, S., ROGLIC, G., GREEN, A., SICREE, R. & KING, H. 2004. Global Prevalence of Diabetes. *Estimates for the year 2000 and projections for 2030,* 27, 1047-1053.

WORLD HEALTH ORGANIZATION. 2014. *Diabetes Key Facts* [Online]. Available: http://www.who.int/en/news-room/fact-sheets/detail/diabetes [Accessed 24 June 2018].

ZUHAID, M., ZAHIR, K. K. & DIJU, I. U. 2012. Knowledge and perceptions of diabetes in urban and semi urban population of Peshawar, Pakistan. *Journal of Ayub Medical College Abbottabad,* 24, 105-108.

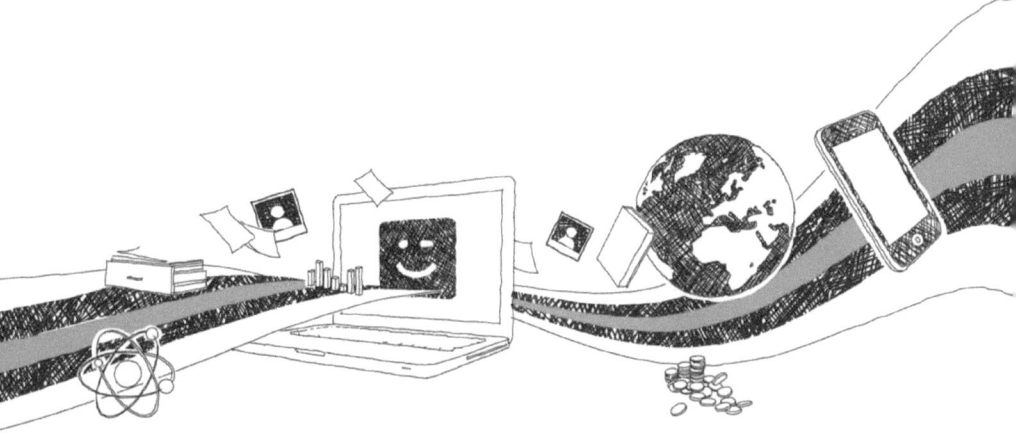
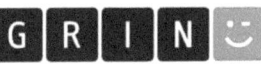